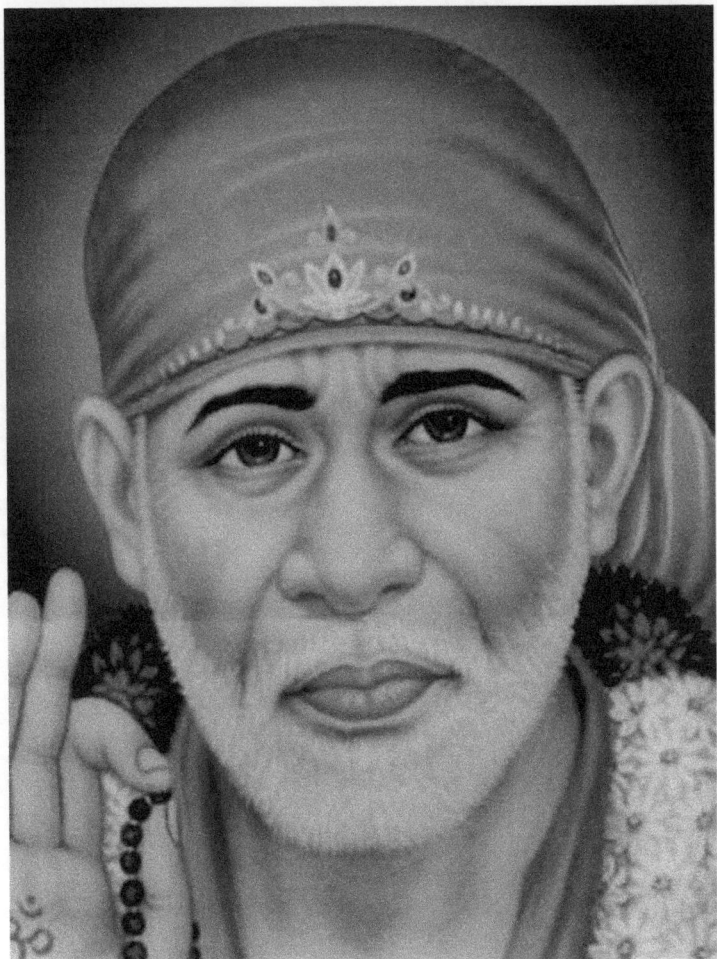

See the Divine in the human being.

Sai Baba of Shirdi

Om Sai Ram

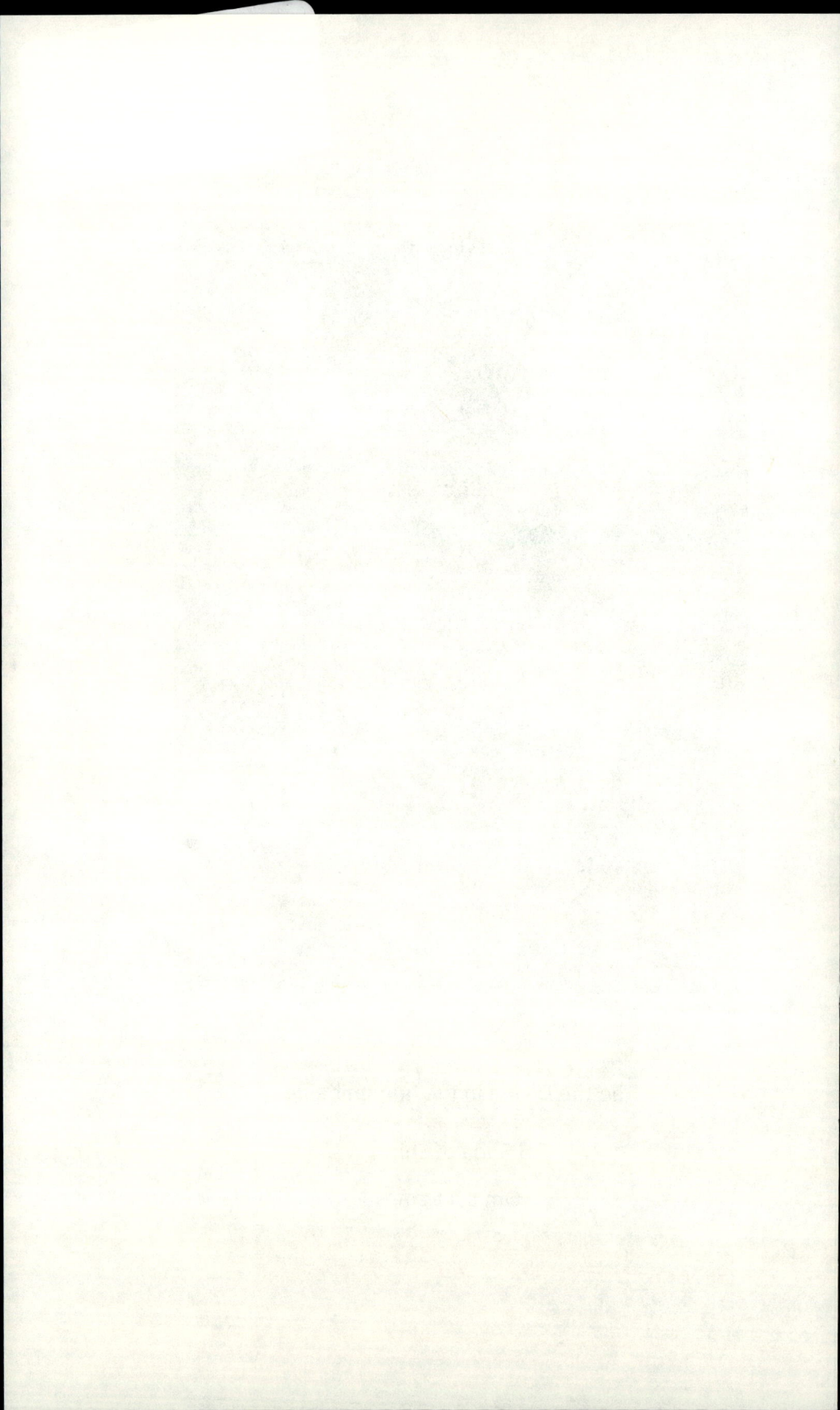

The Lonely Flip Flop

It's never too late to step into
your happy place

POOJA MITTRA

First published by Ultimate World Publishing 2019
Copyright © 2019 Pooja Mittra.

ISBN
Print: 978-1-925884-15-9
Ebook: 978-1-925884-16-6

Cover design: Ultimate World Publishing
Front Cover photograph: SWEviL-Shutterstock.com
Editor: Richard Sine
Typeset and layout: Ultimate World Publishing

ULTIMATE WORLD
—— PUBLISHING ——

Ultimate World Publishing
Diamond Creek,
Victoria Australia 3089
www.writeabook.com.au

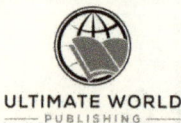

Dedicated to my three birds, for I will raise them to realize

that they are enough, so that one day, they will grow up,

and become unfuckwithable.

Unfuckwithable: Adj. When you're truly at peace and in

touch with yourself; Nothing anyone says or does bothers

you, and no negativity can touch you.

Table of Contents

Part I

The Lonely Flip Flop

EVERYONE'S HAPPY;

FACEBOOK SAYS SO

It's 4 a.m. and I'm driving to the train stop. Next to me sits my <then at the time> husband. He'll leave town for a commute into LA. Night still casts over the skies.

My blinker is on for my right turn. In front of me sits a truck, which is brave enough to turn left without blinking. And, in that moment, it hits me ... I used to be brave, too! I even used to feel invincible! And, I realize, is this my life? Void of any emotions? Any feelings? And maybe the worst is that it's not even painful anymore; like a limb that needs to be amputated, as it no longer serves any purpose to the body, but it still hangs on. It still hangs on, in hopes that it may find its purpose once again.

No, there's a feeling, and it's called hopelessness. A feeling that should be *eradicated* from the face of this earth.

But I'm only 23. This cannot be my story, I think, as tears stream down my face. HONK!! It's my turn to go.

INTUITION: YOUR INNER LIGHTHOUSE

Things will get better. Give it time. You're young. You need to work hard at a marriage. It's not a joke. It's not a *game*! So much advice flooding into my ears – which anyone in their right mind would advise, given that they didn't know the current situation. I know. Nod, nod. Yes. I know. I try to silence the outside noise by agreeing. But my intuition tells me otherwise; it's screaming, "GET OUT! Something isn't right!"

I know that something is not right, but how long do I wait to confirm this? How long is it going to take to have some form of proof, some evidence? I need the evidence so that people will believe me. I just know. My gut knows. <LISTEN

TO YOUR INTUITION. *It's your inner lighthouse.*>

As young girls, we tend to paint a **magical** image of our futures. We set the stage in our minds to be similar to those romantic comedies, where everything is wrapped in a perfect bow at the end of the story. And some people attain this. Well, at least everyone I saw on Facebook was happy: partying, still young, going to grad school, doing something *meaningful*, single, enjoying life … FREE.

I felt such envy. It was a terrible feeling, this *envy*; but it was how I felt in that moment. Why can't people post pictures of their misery? But, more importantly, why do I want others to be unhappy? That's not going to change my situation, and that's just not a nice way of processing my inner feelings. How is it their fault that my life did not take the turn to "happily ever after?" It should *not* make me feel better. That's just not right. I didn't want to feel it, but it just came to me in waves, waves of anger, waves of longing, and waves of hopelessness. I wanted their life. I wanted to jump into the screen and picture myself with my friends, my family, back home, laughing, going back to school. But I made this choice; so, seriously, just deal with it like an adult! I am the only one to blame at this point. Stupid Facebook and its happy drunken free spirits. Bah.

THE FAÇADE

Sunny California – you would think anyone could be happy here. How can someone be in a state of depression *HERE*? The sun was always out to play; I barely felt a rain drop, and there was always something fun happening. People were generally in a good mood; very casual and breezy with their flip flops and "year round good weather" attire.

So, here's the problem: I left my world, my family , friends, and my familiar space for someone who really was able to impress (me) and everyone I knew – the charisma, the charm. *OH MY!* The laughs, the jokes, the mixing and mingling with my loved ones, the FAÇADE, which quickly wore away once we hit the ground on the other side of the country. It was difficult for them to understand my anxiety. How could they possibly understand? *Him*? No ... but he's so charming! How can they believe me, when I, MYSELF, could hardly believe it? How could I explain that things were so different?

How could I explain to them that during our honeymoon, he stood outside of the temple and refused to come inside as I walked in alone. And just a few months before, my family and friends witnessed him attend ALL of the religious ceremonies in the temple and participate in *ALL* of the rituals with a smile plastered on his face. That was a PRE-wedding show. It was an Oscar-worthy performance.

How could I explain to people that I was asked to remove a photo of Sai Baba of Shirdi (a saint who I grew up following and continue to follow today) from the fireplace mantel, because he was ashamed at what our guests would think. That photo was one of the few meaningful connections I had with my childhood, and I am still so angry at myself for taking it down from the mantel. That's where I've seen it, front and center, my whole life. But I took it down because someone else was ashamed of it being there.

THE "NOT ENOUGH" FALLACY

We often wonder why people stay in a broken, stale relationship. "What's wrong with them? Why can't they just get out of it?" On the outside it seems so obvious: a simple solution is to just get out, move on, find someone else. "Don't you have any self-respect?"

But there are so many reasons one may have, not just one or two reasons. It can be so complex to the point that the person IN IT cannot even answer that question. Is it the fear of being alone, or the fear of being unable to find someone when all of this is over? Is it the fear of having that uncomfortable conversation? Or, is it the fear of what others around you will think or say about you? Our mind goes into a downward spiral before we even have a chance to think straight. "If I leave this relationship, everyone around me will start rumors and say really terrible things about me and my family; then word will get around, and no one will want to engage in a relationship with me. I will never get married again or have children. I will die alone." Boom! We create our own misery in our minds that hasn't even *happened*. Those are pretty intense and gloomy thoughts that we set ourselves up to believe. So, what do we do? Do we stay and suffer it out? OR, do we conquer the thoughts that have NOT EVEN happened, and rise above? I think we all know that the heart wants the latter, but the mind plays tricks on us, convincing us that the comfortable and safe play is best.

We may think that we are not enough, or not good enough. This is a very deep-rooted philosophy that is anchored in some of us – maybe from childhood. We may feel that we are not enough, therefore we do not deserve the good things that life has to offer because someone may have told us this at some point in our lives. And, from that moment forward, we formulated our truth around their baseless assumption of who we are.

KNOB (SNOB) HILL

Knob Hill (or *Snob Hill,* as some called it) was the name of the neighborhood that we had moved into when my dad rose up to a higher position in the company for which he was working, and was able to afford a beautiful three-story brick house in Rocky Mount, North Carolina, with two Mercedes Benz lounging in the driveway. We had a variety of fruit trees in the backyard. The long driveway had an artery that split the front yard into two sections and created a walkway to a porch leading to the front door. It was a neighborhood and community where everyone knew each other.

We were also the *only* South Asian family in that community at the time. The only family who made their guests remove their shoes before entering their home – which was such a foreign concept to my friends, who came over often and would giggle when they saw the "Thanks for Taking Your Shoes Off" sign at the front door. I'll never forget that sign, which was printed out using Microsoft Word and had a border of feet all around; attached to the door with Scotch tape. And now it is a common practice; most people appreciate the fact that you take your shoes off when entering their homes, for obvious and hygienic reasons. The Eastern philosophies and traditions always tend to catch on in Western society.

We had missionaries ring our doorbell, dressed in nice suits and ties, Bible in one hand, trying to guide us to follow their truth. They thought that they were doing the right thing, trying to spread the word of God to us, trying to "save" us. It was almost a once-a-month check in with house #613 on Nichole Lane. Hmmm.. Let's see if they're 'down' with Christianity today. Those poor chaps, left with their head hanging each time, Bible in one hand. My parents graciously declined their every visit.

We finally had what my parents had moved here for, but did we really? It still felt like we did not fit in. *And we didn't.*

In the beginning of the school year (I was in sixth grade, I believe) a local country club representative went to everyone's home to see who wanted to enroll in a cotillion program, a program that blended various types of ballroom dancing with classes in table etiquette and how to be respectful and polite to members of their communities. I would listen to all my friends talking and laughing about how much fun they had at that class. They had a bunch "of "inside stories and jokes,: all relating to their lessons, jokes about the instructors etc.. Somehow the representative skipped over our house, and we were not invited to be a part of that "society." Is etiquette only reserved for certain people? I had nothing to contribute, but I would listen, and wonder why house #613 was always skipped, year after year.

It was a Saturday afternoon. I was sitting on the bed at a friend's home in my neighborhood when she and another friend came and sat right next to me. I looked at them like they were acting a bit weird, and they were not smiling. They wore very serious expressions on their faces, which told me that they may have something important to tell me. One of the girls took my hands, and looked at me in the eyes, and said, "Pooja, we are really worried about you. We think that you and your family are going to hell, because you don't believe in Jesus Christ."

You know that moment when you're in total shock and you basically cannot formulate a proper sentence because the thoughts in your mind are incoherent? An uncomfortable heat sensation began to rise into my chest and managed to sneak its way up to my ears. I was eleven. And I went home in tears, angry; not at them, but at my parents -because we had the wrong religion. I was not good enough to go to heaven. That's why I wasn't chosen to be in that cotillion. That's why I'm going to hell, along with my family. Everything was coming together. And from these small experiences growing up (there are more), that ridiculous belief and feeling of being inadequate stayed with me for many, many years. At the time, you feel the hurt, and eventually move on, because you cannot dwell on them forever. But they somehow sneak back into your life later on, if they go unresolved. You end up somewhere along the lines, choosing a profession, or choosing a partner, based on a perception of yourself that was cast

upon you during your childhood because you may not

believe that you deserve better.

ROOMIES

Now going back into the future to Cali. I used to joke about being a "roommate," but that joke was my reality. The joke was on ME. I approached the subject several times, but each time it was casually brushed off. For almost three years, I seriously thought that something was wrong with ME. Why does my husband not 'want' me? Why does he deliberately keep himself distant? Was I not pretty enough, funny enough, loveable enough; so what is it? This was the most embarrassing fact I eventually had to break to my parents. And I hate that I was put in that position, because we don't discuss *those* things. During our childhood, my sister and I would pretend that we had to go to the bathroom if a kissing scene came up in a movie, so you can only imagine the shame I felt when I had to share my truth. Toward the latter part of my time there, I started to sleep in our guest room. Either way, it made no difference.

DISTRACT AND DEFLECT

VIZUALIZE: Being back with the family, laughing so hard with my mom over something we couldn't even explain until we had tears in our eyes. We always did that. Everyone else would join in on the laughter, not even knowing what it was about. And at times, we didn't even know. But it was so much fun.

Sitting at the kitchen island with mom, having a cup of Darjeeling tea; that fresh smell and the heat that hits your face once you take a sip. Classic Bollywood songs from the 60s play in the background, while we chat, and laugh and chat some more. Dad walks in and pretends to be busy doing something, but he is secretly listening to our conversation as he wants to be a part of the fun. Oh, I miss it. I want to have tea with her every day. Such simple days. Such simple love.

Reality sets in. Wake up. I am here, not there. I start taking courses in interior design. I love interior décor, design, anything to do with decorating. There's a community college just a few miles down from where I work as an engineer (I really hated engineering and was terrible at it); so this new community college became a haven of temporary relief. I loved those two hours I was learning about something I enjoyed. And, more importantly, it saved me from going back home, which meant less time with him. <ESCAPING FROM REALITY is a temporary solution. *It solves nothing*. Confront the uncomfortable. Solutions only arise by confrontation. It's easy to avoid

those awkward conversations, but having them makes us

much stronger>

NO THANK YOU

The beautiful seasons of Virginia; the lightning bugs that lit up summer evenings; the faint sun during the fall that gently kissed the trees and turned them into gorgeous shades of burgundy, gold and orange; and those air-crisp nights during the winters that we would spend by the fireplace. Maybe I wouldn't miss it so much if I were at peace here. I have nothing. I want to go home. I am unwanted, like a piece of furniture that was once so impressive, but lost its shine and waits in the corner for some company.

"Here's your prescription for Klonopin. It will act as a sedative and help you with your anxiety and panic attacks." Oh, thank you, Doctor. A relaxed state of mind sets in, movements are slower. This wonder pill is creating a fake feeling for me so that I can get through the days. So now, this once, lively personality full of positivity, relies on a white pill to thrive.? My happiness depends on this medication? This is not my life. I won't allow it! I am determined not to fall into the trap of medication. Prescription goes into the trash. Good bye, Klonopin, it was nice knowing you for two weeks of my life. I'm going to be happy! Whatever it takes. I am not going to rely on medication to be happy. Deep down, I know this is not a neurological issue, it's definitely a situation-based depression, and I can always change my situation. Anyone can.

THE LONELY FLIP FLOP

My eyes are open as I lay on my bed. I see a lonely flip flop on the roof of a shed next door. It's been there for months, and I always wonder how it got there. No one even bothers to remove it; maybe they don't even know it's up there. I can see it from the second floor of my house. There was just one flip flop.

I felt like I could relate. It was supposed to be a pair.

OMG. I am that flip flop. Am I going crazy?

Sometimes it's better to be a lonely flip flop rather than be paired with one that's the wrong size.

VISUALIZE. I'm back East, and feel so happy at home, at peace with people who know me, who love me, and want to be around me. Why do I crave to be wanted and loved? Because that's what humans do. We flourish off of that feeling. Isn't it natural?

 I can smell the chicken curry that my mom cooks on the stove; the strong aroma of ginger, garlic, and onions, simmering, doing a little happy dance as they heat up in the oil.

She's a life-long vegetarian, but cooks meat for my dad, because he enjoys it. That's love:-wanting to make the other person happy because it makes YOU happy to see THEM happy. Why is that concept so difficult?

I open my eyes and I see him flexing his muscles in the mirror and staring at progress. He's moving forward. He's developing muscles. Why? The endless hours at the gym

are for whom? –obviously for the reflection in the mirror.

I'm watching from the background, as my eyes roll to the

back of my head.

THE BUFFER EFFECT

I owe my sanity to my coworkers. Even though my job was definitely not my dream job, the people there were like instant family. If only they could change my personal situation ... I wanted to pack them in a box and bring them home, so I had a buffer. Why do I need a buffer? I have tried talking — starting a conversation about our relationship — several times, even suggested counseling; but no remedy, no course of action, nothing was taken seriously. Am I out of options? We can sit in the car for hours in silence. Show up to people's events and he turns into a complete showman- WOW. Where did that come from? Who are you? Do I know you? We host parties, and drinks are being made, friends are having fun- laughing and joking- and he's hosting like he's going to win an award. They all leave. Doors close. Separate rooms. Go to sleep. People would NEVER know. This is not my story! This will not be my story. Not MY life.

The garage door opens after a long day at work. Oh, no. Today is not gym day. I run upstairs and go for a long bath. Maybe something will happen tonight? Wishful thinking. I'm not worth it. Something is wrong with me. I don't know what it is, but obviously something must be wrong with me when my spouse has been keeping his distance from me for almost three years. So the depression sets in.

Neglect is a form of abuse that creeps up slowly on you, like one too many Sambuca's—so smooth, you don't even know what hit you.

I am late for work on most days. I don't want get out of bed. Where do I go? Who do I talk to? Who do I even tell, and will they believe me? I eat. And eat. 25 pounds gained. Just like that. It feels good to indulge. And it doesn't matter.

NAMASTEY, INDIA

My parents plan a trip to India — an annual trip — to volunteer at the eye camp, which is a team of amazing, selfless people (doctors and volunteers) who together join efforts to orchestrate the organization of the camp — from registering the patients, to having them screened by doctors, providing food and lodging for them, administer the cataract surgeries if needed, and provide post-operative care. For three days, we did just that.

I learned that there is SO much more to life than just my sob story. There are things we can do to help other people. There is a whole world of people who need uplifting in different ways. My mom and I laughed and joked with the women there, who insisted that we take their photos while they struck a pose; after the photo, they would run to our side to see the drama unfold and giggle. We danced with them. We listened to their stories. It was truly amazing.

Being involved with the eyecamp was something I wanted to do without anything in return; however, I failed. I left there with a new perspective. They gave me a new way of thinking. I wasn't helping these poor villagers. Not at all. They were helping me. They were opening MY eyes and allowing me to serve them, and to understand that we have so much of ourselves to offer to others. All this time I was so wrapped up in myself, my feelings, my situation — something from which I can easily remove myself; so consumed in my own set of problems.

I had not been so genuinely happy in so long.

While away, I was able to THINK about what I wanted. I didn't miss him, not one bit! Nor did he miss me. I may have gotten one or two messages from him the entire trip. This is not how it was supposed to be, but it's OKAY.

I would rather the truth be displayed rather than phony displays of affection.

For the first time in a very long time, I felt like me. It is always a good idea to take some time off and be away. Your mind cannot come to any realizations when you're IN IT ... so take some time off, and give yourself space to think, and to feel. Sometimes, you don't have to feel *anything*, and that's when you know.

I have everything: a supportive family and the means to CHOOSE my happiness. I am not stuck. I can be happy. I WILL be happy.

I told mom everything at Heathrow Airport. Cried and cried to her on the way home. All of my bottled up emotions and anger came out, and she was there, listening without judgement, as she always does. We were together up until London, and then she was off to DC, and I was off to LA. But after almost three years of this hopeless feeling, I was finally, finally able to break the silence, and release all of the negative feelings and emotions to one of the most entrusted people in my life: my mom.

THE WISE COOKIE

Over the next two months I unraveled. I was determined that this is not going to be my story. I knew that if I walked out that door, there would be no effect on the other side. So, what's my purpose here? Am I going to be sad and depressed, and just ride out the rest of my life like this? That will not be my story. I won't allow it! I choose my happiness. I choose my state of mind.

Get up! Get dressed! YES! Today, I choose to be happy. I will find my happiness. I will get out. I will leave. I am DONE. I took myself on a date to the Chinese restaurant across the street. <A date with yourself is CRUCIAL. Sad,

happy, nervous, whatever state of mind you are in. Take yourself on a date. Reconnect and think about what you want, or think about all the things for which you are grateful>

The fortune cookie cracked open "You made the right choice." Tears flow. I believe in signs. I swear, this is no joke; I know some may be laughing, but the universe sends signals. I FELT my signal. I made the choice to be happy, and the fortune cookie is on board and on point.

With the help and support of my parents, my sister, and my best friends, I was able to rise up.

I wanted to secure a job before physically moving. "You're lucky if you find something at $50K with your credentials," his voice echoed in my ears. That was my worth. He *TOLD* me, didn't he? "You need to accept that you leave everything and move with your partner. You're a woman.

You get the short end of the stick. Accept it."

I don't need to "accept" ANYTHING, I thought to myself.

The feeling of emotional freedom was awesome, and I was

on a high. Nothing could be said to upset me.

FLY AWAY

Dad picked me up from the airport to take me to my interview. "Are you sure about this?" Yes, 100%. I had one interview for an engineering position that was ten minutes away from my parents' house. One interview, 3,000 miles away. Dear Sai Baba, if I get this job, that means I am making the right choice. I STILL needed the validation that I'm doing the right thing. This was the biggest decision in my life! One of the biggest decisions I had ever made. Divorce was such a taboo in my community. Forget those people who judge. What do *they* know? I'll just be a hot topic for a few days. This is my LIFE. I need to fix it. I need a detour so that the next chapter can be positive. I'm not going to allow my story to become one sad sob story, and mope around. Enough moping around. Enough is enough.

I got the job. And it paid $55k. "So THERE!" is what I wanted to say.

And that's how I slowly lifted myself up. With an "enough is enough" attitude.

My one way ticket is booked. Everything is packed, with the help of my Dad. And shipped back East.

My dad. My savior. It was an awkward moment for him. He had to see his own mother struggle, but he vowed *never* to allow his daughters to struggle. He made sure we could stand on our own two feet. That's why he pushed for the engineering and the medical professions for my sister and me. People would judge, but he knew what he was doing. He didn't care what others said. He never did.

He is a maverick. Of his own mind. And he pushed us toward these professions in his own right. His motivation for guiding us into these professions was never to show off to others; he's not that type. He simply wanted my sister and I to be able to have a solid degree, so that we could be financially secure should we face hardships in the future. And maybe it's because of him that I was able to get that job after ONE interview. I owe him. Big time. Even today, as I follow my passion as an interior and event decorator, he is by my side ... always supportive.

Dad tried to reason with him to see if there was any chance that the relationship could be mended; after the conversation he told me that he would support me either way, and that the decision was mine.

Dad left after helping me pack. I dropped him to LAX, "See you in two weeks, Dad."

NIMA THE GREAT

I couldn't stay in that house knowing I was about to leave. It was all too awkward. My work friend, who became a sister to me (let's call her a disguised name: Nima) took me in her home to stay with her. Before leaving he asks,

HIM: How are you going to get there <Nima's house>

ME: Drive

HIM: Who's car are you going to take. That's not your car to drive. (his parents, whom I really adored, gave me their old Infinity when I had moved there. I would sometimes go straight to their house after work to hang out with them and have tea. They were very kind hearted. But, at the end of the day, I was not married to THEM.)

Nima came to pick me up while he was at work. We cleaned the whole house. She gave me the best advice. "Leave with dignity." Together we scrubbed the bathroom floors, vacuumed, mopped, dusted, and done. The house was clean and spotless. She took me to the carwash to get the car cleaned. She had major anxiety while being in that carwash as she suffered from claustrophobia, but she sat with me during the carwash. And we laughed, because I knew she wanted to jump out of the car. We always had so much fun together. She was like an older sister to me.

Cleaned, washed, and vacuumed. We then returned to the house, I dropped the newly cleaned car and the keys. On the way out, I tossed the wedding albums into the trash. I was relieved, angry, sad. Every emotion that I could imagine. He didn't try to stop me. I stayed at Nima's home

for about one week. He knew where she lived, but didn't

try to come over and stop me (like in the movies). Maybe

this is what he secretly wanted; maybe he wanted out as

much as I did, and this was his way of opening the door for

me. A door to a better life, for the both of us.

Today, I am thankful to him for guiding me to that door.

Because behind that door was a whole new world, a world

of unstoppable happiness, that was waiting to receive me.

THE ART OF VISUALIZATION

VISUALIZATION. Where do I want to be? With whom do I want to spend my days laughing? I love to laugh. I love ridiculous jokes. I see happiness. I see people who I love to be around. I used to spend so much time just visualizing a reality that I wanted so badly.

Now, thirteen years later, I find out that there is something called "creative visualization," which is a method used to take you where you want to be in life. Practice for a few moments a day, just visualizing. It's an art. I remember doing just that during those miserable years, and I had no idea that it was an actual practice.

It made me feel so good – to put those thoughts out there in the universe, and, in turn, I swear, the universe sent me signs, and angels in the form of people who helped me. I was able to attain this "enough is enough" attitude, get up, and get OUT of it, all with the support of loved ones, to who I am forever in debt.

The more you think about where you want to be, the more you obsess (in a good way) about it, your mind and body will start to act accordingly. Connections will be made. But this is ONLY if it's a genuine want, a true longing. Like you cannot imagine your life ANY other way.

GET YOUR HAPPY ON

I say this to any man or woman in a broken relationship. Sometimes it just cannot be fixed. Sometimes there is not an answer to why it is falling apart. Do you spend your remaining years living a lie?

Both parties are being unfair to one another, robbing one another of a happiness that could be experienced.

No, relationships are not easy. I do not want to give off the impression that you should not even TRY. But after all attempts have been made to mend a broken relationship, after you have possibly given it your all, and still things are not unfolding as desired, then it's really time to move on! Break each other free of the unhappy cycle.

There will be emotional tornados and hurricanes and earthquakes and torrential rainstorms, but if someone is willing to be right there with you to pick up the debris after the storm, and eventually laugh it off (one day), someone who you could not imagine each passing day without, someone with whom you could have fun at 4 a.m. while waiting in line in the grocery store, someone who talks to you on your entire drive home because they know you're exhausted and want to make sure you don't fall asleep behind the wheel, someone who actually knows what you're thinking or about to say just by your expressions, someone who loves you for your flaws and weaknesses, someone who doesn't hold your past against you, someone who treats you with the utmost respect (and vice versa), someone who never judges or questions decisions that mean the world to you, someone who supports you and pushes you to be the BEST version of yourself that you can be, someone who helps you to realize your purpose on this earth, and someone whom you can TRULY call your best friend, you've found your gold.

After I left California, it took me eight years and a couple of unstable relationships to discover my pot of gold, but I just knew it was there. I found my inner strength through the journey that lead me to where I needed to be. There are no regrets over mistakes made during that phase, because each mistake guided me to the right place.

I started writing this as bullet points of my experiences and feelings during those years; for so long I wanted to erase it somehow, just get rid of those terrible memories! I just wanted to leave that part of my life behind. But now I want to remember each day and each feeling that was felt; not because I want to be depressed about it — quite the opposite. The more I remember those times, the more I am grateful and thankful for each day that I am experiencing today.

Today, as I stare at my kids giggling and sitting on top of my husband while they sing along to Despacito in our living room, I know that the choice I made about ten years ago, was the RIGHT one. There is no question about it.

If you find yourself in a bad place, know that there is a way out. Even during the most hopeless of situations, it may seem as if an impending doom is looming over you like a storm cloud on the verge of erupting into a rain shower. Sometimes a good storm knocks at your door just to clear the pathway; at the time we just do not see it that way. If you just allow yourself to change your mindset, and refuse to let this feeling overcome you, there IS happiness. Realize your own worth and what you have to offer, without giving anyone the liberty of defining your importance. You choose your own path to happiness. You write your own story. Happiness lies within all of us. We just have to be brave enough to define it, own it, and conquer it.

PART II

LET'S GET HAPPY

It truly sucks to be in a bad situation, and you're told to find your happiness ... but how? What are some steps you can take that will move you toward the direction of living a peaceful and more fulfilled life? There will be no such situation as a problem-free one, but you will understand how to DEAL with them, when they arise, instead of harping on problems and visualizing an impending doom – like situation ahead.

WE TEACH PEAPLE HOW TO TREAT US

I would strongly suggest to begin with the way you treat yourself and the way you allow others to treat you. This would be the first step toward making peace with yourself.

We cannot expect others to love and respect us, if we do not have those feelings toward ourselves. WE CANNOT EXPECT OTHERS TO LOVE AND RESPECT US, IF WE DO NOT HAVE THOSE FEELINGS TOWARD OURSELVES.

We *teach* people how to *treat* us. If we condone disrespect and hurtful behavior toward us, we cannot blame the other person. We need to set limits as to how we treat ourselves and how we allow others to treat us. This is a crucial first step in ANY relationship, and it starts with the relationship that we have with ourselves. Let go of the people who bring you down until they are able understand that their behavior is unacceptable; and if they cannot find it within themselves to change their attitude, *is your relationship with them really worth it?*

Surround yourself with people who are uplifting. It's time to say GOODBYE to the gray clouds in your life because they are not good for your well-being. Maybe someday when you are at your highest levels of internal happiness, you can stop by and give them a lift. But, for now, focus on you, and focus on getting out of the slump. Everyone has been there at some point, whether he/she admits it or not. And everyone is able to get out of it, too; that is, if they have the will and the hunger to be happy.

WHAT YOU THINK,

YOU BECOME ~ BUDDHA

Negative self-talk is one of the main causes of depression. It's that voice in our head that belittles, judges, and says hurtful things to our spirit. "I'm such a moron ... how could I make such a stupid mistake? I hate myself.; I look disgusting>; Why would anyone want to go on a date with me, I'm such a loser?" and so on.

Ask yourself, *would you say these terrible things to someone else*?

We try to be on our best behavior and treat others nicely and with respect. We conduct ourselves cordially when in social settings or when in someone else's home.

But what about the most important space in our lives? The space we reside in every day. What about our internal home, our brains, our hearts? We brush our teeth, comb our hair, shower, and keep up with our physical hygiene; but what about our mental hygiene?

This is our first home, and we cannot outsource housekeeping. We need to do it ourselves. So, then, why do we reserve the nice comments for others?

When you constantly tell yourself such limiting and demoralizing beliefs, it becomes habitual … and we are creatures of habit. What happens next? You begin truly to believe these things; then this changes your self-image. It's a downward spiral from there. We will then act according to what we believe, and will take steps in the direction that will further confirm this negative inner voice. The mind is a powerful tool with which we have been gifted. Unfortunately, if we use it the wrong way, it can be harmful to our well-being. Studies have proven that these mean and bullying thoughts directly affect your breathing rate, heart rate, and blood pressure! So these thoughts are not just harmful to your mind, but to your body as well.

Now imagine if we shifted our beliefs and told ourselves UPLIFTING things! How do we do this?

Every day, make it a point to say something nice to yourself, OUT LOUD. Comment on yourself positively, both for your physical appearance and your emotional state of mind and being. Think about the type of person you WANT to be. Focus on traits that you admire and respect – *write it out*. And tell yourself that you are those things. Even if that inner critic in you is trying to shut you down, just keep talking over that voice and internalize the person you want to be. Do this exercise daily, when you have a few minutes to spare, or when you feel that the "downer voice" in your mind is overwhelming. Separate that voice from yourself. That voice was constructed. It could be from influences outside of your control (expectations from others such as parents, bosses, etc.).

We are taught to be tough on ourselves- we are taught to not "toot our horns."

TOOT YOUR HORN, <in a good, healthy way>.

Be kinder to yourself.

Delete negative self-talk. Just take it out of your system. We beat ourselves up over a mistake, or something we may have said that was stupid. It's OK. At the end of the day, if you feel that your action or words emotionally hurt someone, pick up the phone or meet that individual in

person, and let them know that you are genuinely sorry.
Don't agonize over things said or done for days; if
something is bothering you, just take action and do
something to rectify it. Write it out first. Clear your
thoughts, get out a pen and paper and WRITE. Sometimes
just writing things out can help resolve your emotions. If
you need to talk it out, confide in someone you trust and
someone who does not judge you. We all make mistakes.
This is why we are human. We just *deal* with them
differently.

Own up to your mistake, offer a genuine apology, make a
conscious effort to not repeat it, and MOVE FORWARD. Do
not dwell on mistakes. Mistakes are gurus. They help us to
learn and grow, and eventually will lead us to the right
direction and to the kind of person we aim to be.

Select your five favorite traits in people you admire, and every day say that you are those things OUT LOUD and IN FRONT of the mirror – once when you wake up and once before going to bed. For example, "I am strong, I am brave, I am kind, I am compassionate, I am smart." When you say them, BELIEVE them. And knock out the conflicting thoughts.

So I will take this opportunity to assist in any way possible for you to avoid putting this exercise off for some other time. Let's select five words. I'll fill in the first one, because every person should wake up feeling and knowing that he or she is ENOUGH. Grab a pen and choose the next four words that you will say to yourself every day:

I AM:

1. ENOUGH

2.

3.

4.

5.

The more love you give to yourself, the more you will have

to offer to others.

CULTURAL TABOOS

They just need to go away. This is a topic that is so ridiculous but so relevant. It doesn't matter what decade you're in, these "taboos" follow you wherever you go. And it's the small minded people who fall prey to them who keep these taboos alive.

I can speak, for sure, for my cultural background: South Asian. A big taboo is divorce. And it's usually (not always) worse when the woman decides to leave the marriage. Society is SO wrapped up in what others are going to think that people will actually live their lives to gain the approval of others, or, even WORSE, parents pressure their kids to be a certain way, excel in certain fields (i.e., medicine, engineering, or law – of course, because those are the only professions that exist, right?), or pressure their kids to STAY in a broken marriage in an effort to avoid shame on the family, or to avoid the gossip that will follow.

So. if you really break it down, a parent would actually WANT their child to SUFFER and be MISERABLE for the rest of his/her lives, just so they can get some kind of applause from an audience who doesn't really matter; to an audience who will probably talk smack either way; to an audience who may even gloat in the grief of others. For what? Who MATTERS at the end of the day? Why can't we think about what we are doing to our own loved ones? We need to allow our loved ones to find their happiness.

It's so arrogant to intercept another person's quest for happiness just to satisfy your own cravings. That person can be your child, your best friend, your mother, your sister. If you truly want other humans to blossom, let them be. Let them figure it out.

Luckily, I come from a nontraditional family; my parents align themselves with traditional values and modern thought. When I finally had the courage to lay out my story, they said,"' Whatever you decide, we support you."

A lot of women are not that lucky, especially in my culture. Once they get married, their parents close their doors. That's it. You "belong" to your husband's family. Make it work. Regardless of how your life is going to be, *make* it work. This is the part where BOTH sides need to listen, loud and clear. Parents should support their daughters and sons if they are going through a rough marriage. No one should be compelled to tolerate any abuse, be it emotional or physical. Who CARES what people think? WHO CARES WHAT PEOPLE THINK?

Once you start living for society, you may as well stop living. Why are you trying to live someone else's life? Do you really think those who pass judgment are living an ideal life? Who are THEY to point fingers? This seems to be COMMON SENSE. But it's NOT. It needs to be spelled out and pasted everywhere. WHO CARES WHAT PEOPLE THINK? Choose your own happiness. This is NOT selfish, this is YOUR life. How do you want your story to play out? How do you envision your life to be? If your current situation is not aligned with HOW you visualize yourself in the future, something needs to change. And if you need to remove some negative factors (people) in your life to do so, then that's just what you need to do.

Is it easy? Hell no. But ease will never please, my friend. It's the struggle, the fight, the painful truth, that will eventually set you free to the person you would like to be.

It's about time we stop trying to prove ourselves and start IMPROVING ourselves to be the best. Living someone else's dream is a lie. It's a bubble in which you will float around until you realize, one day, after drifting off so far from YOUR OWN dream – POP! It bursts. What are you to do at that point? It may be too late? You may be 75 years old and have truly lived a life that you regret.

OR, you can take control of your life, understand what it is you truly love and want; what drives YOU, what gives you that ammunition when you talk about "it," and create your own bubble. Drift off into your own element.

Don't assume that everything is hunky dory because of how people appear. People want to put on a facade to make it seem like their lives are perfect. No one knows what goes on in private.

If you're "that couple," it will get exhausting to keep wearing the mask with a smile plastered on your faces. This lifestyle will just make you bitter and cynical into your old age. We spend way too much time, money, and effort trying to appear a certain way for OTHER people. If they're going to judge you, are they really worth your time?

We are so wired to be in tune with how others will judge us – so much that we become deaf to what WE want.

What WE want is really what THEY expect. How ASSbackwards is that? If you're doing that... just stop.

From this point onward, STOP. It's not too late. <DJ stop

the music.>

Start dancing to your own fucking tune.

EMOTIONAL ABUSE & NEGLECT

I felt ugly and untouchable.

I felt ashamed because I wanted the intimacy with my husband during those years.

I felt embarrassed because I had to ask for what should have been a natural occurrence for a couple, and was rejected each time.

I felt angry because I waited until I got married, and THIS was the result.

I felt humiliated because I was told by him that there's more to a marriage than intimacy.

I felt confused because I was told that "things slow down when you're in your 30s."

I felt inadequate when I was told that his energy had to be saved for the gym.

And I felt like sinking into the floor when my dad asked him "why," and his answer was that I was "boring."

Dejected, rejected and confused was my state of being. I was just there to pass the days, floating around in a world void of emotion and physical connection. The worst part was that I didn't even know why. There was no reason for this behavior. It was totally perplexing. And, to this day, I still don't know why as I can only suspect.

That feeling of utter rejection was my rock bottom, but it somehow gave me this rush of energy to get out. That feeling gave me insight as to what I want out of life, because I now had a bitter taste of what I will never choose to accept again.

Recognize it. Abuse is not always physical.

Emotional abuse is doing things to someone that can be hurtful and traumatizing. Emotional neglect is failing to do things that will help promote the emotional well-being of another.

It's very confusing to be the target in such a situation, because you don't understand how to react. It's not black or white. You're not being physically harmed. However, the emotional scarring that can result when you're at the receiving end of it is, without a doubt, difficult to recover from.

When your partner prefers to spend time alone engaging in activities such as going to the gym, refusing to spend time with their significant other, not engaging in conversation, avoiding and making excuses for intimacy, the list goes on—this is emotional neglect, and, over time, can really hamper the self-esteem and self-worth of his/her partner.

See the signs. If you're not sure, create a journal of the days you felt emotionally neglected and what the causes may have been. When you're in it," it's difficult to see, and sadly you become used to that behavior. Never allow anyone to belittle you or make you feel like you don't matter.

It's a terrible feeling, and creating a log will help you to understand the situation more clearly, instead of having random thoughts and occurrences floating around in your mind. Get organized and assess your relationship and how you wish to be treated. If there is a disconnect between your actual relationship and how you wish to be treated, then share your concerns with your partner. Create a list of your expectations of how your partner should be emotionally and physically supportive. What are some of the behaviors you consider when you think of an emotionally and physically supportive partner? Now make a list of what you're currently experiencing and see how they compare.

Also, it's important to examine your own behavior. Are you doing your part to create a healthy relationship? And this needs to be an honest assessment - no one is reading this but you. What are some things that you are doing or could be doing to strengthen the bond between you both?

If you have honestly done this exercise, and shared your concerns with your partner, and there is still an awkwardness between you both, then seek professional counseling as the next step.

Do what you need to do to make your life not *just* livable, but ENJOYABLE.

ME-TIME

Take yourself on a date at least once in two weeks. Go to your favorite restaurant, order your favorite meal, and enjoy a date with yourself. As a mom of three tiny children, (2-year-old twins and a 4-year-old), I take myself out. I enjoy a nice HOT meal. (Usually by the time I eat, my food is cold, or I end up eating leftovers from their plates and call it a day). So I enjoy MY time alone, while I contemplate life and all the things for which I am grateful, and think about how I can improve as a mother, wife, daughter, and just as a human being. Sometimes I bring a small journal with me and write it out, so that these thoughts become more real. I am constantly trying to learn and improve, and this is what gives me hope to move forward in life.

So, carve out some time, even if it's just 30 minutes once in two weeks, to take yourself out to lunch. It doesn't have to be a fancy restaurant with valet parking. Go to Chipotle. Just order your food, sit at a table, and enjoy those quiet moments with yourself. If you have more time, go see a movie with yourself. People freak out at the notion of going places and sitting ... why? Why are we afraid to be alone with ourselves? Self-connection is key to having healthy relationships OUTSIDE of the one you have with yourself. If YOU don't know YOU, then how do you expect other people to know YOU? If you are not comfortable spending time with YOU, then how can others feel comfortable spending time with YOU?

BREATH IN THE MOMENT

Meditation is an ancient practice, and it has been scientifically proven to reduce and even eliminate anxiety, improve sleep, increase focus, and strengthen personal relationships. This simple routine, if incorporated, will be life changing to you and for the people around you. Meditation will allow you to enhance several facets of your human existence, such as health, energy levels, performance, and happiness. I personally wish that I had started earlier in my life; but it's never too late to incorporate the practice of meditation into your own life. And, with today's technology, we have tutorials and guides at our fingertips: YouTube, podcasts, you name it. So, it would behoove you to educate yourself on this topic and include it in your daily routine. There are unlimited resources to help guide you on this hot practice, and there are many different types. Do a little research as to which type of meditation technique works best for you.

Boxed breathing is a breathing technique I have been using for some time now; it helps me to focus and de-stress. It's very simple. Breathe in for 4 seconds, hold your breath for 4 seconds, breathe out for 4 seconds, and hold your breath for 4 seconds. Repeat. You are creating a virtual box with your breathing. It's easy and can be done anywhere.

INVITE YOUR DESIRED REALITY

This is, hands down, one of my favorite experiences; it may seem a little crazy when you first encounter it. Your mind is so powerful that it can literally alter your reality. If you sit down and really think about it, the concept is logical. Visualize where you want to be in a certain amount of time – it could be 6 months, 1 year, 3 years, or so on. Visualize it in absolute detail. Close your eyes and listen to the sounds you want to hear, the smells you want to smell, the way you would like to present yourself, and how this new "life" will contribute to you, your loved ones, and to the well-being of others. Do this exercise for just a few minutes every day; and, if you genuinely believe in what you are envisioning, your body and mind will take the necessary steps to get to that point. As you obsess over it<in a healthy way>, you are sending signals out into the universe, and, in turn, the universe will send you signs, signals, and people who will help you reach your goals. You just have to believe in it, and believe in it strongly.

CONTRIBUTION

Contribution is powerful. As humans, we are naturally built to want to help others. We all have a sense of compassion and a sense of purpose. If you find yourself wanting to make a positive difference in the life of another, then make some phone calls, meet with people who are able to help you do this, and do it. There is no better feeling than coming to the aid of someone who needs it. It could be visiting senior citizens at their homes and playing games or reading to them; it could be visiting patients in the hospital, providing school supplies to children who cannot afford them, etc. Whatever cause "hits home" to you — that's the one. Studies have shown that when people contribute to society in a positive way, it activates regions of the brain that are connected to pleasure and trust. Altruistic behavior is also known to release endorphins in the brain. This is a wonderful way to connect with other people and release more compassion and humanity into the world, of which there is never a shortage.

THE SPICES OF LIFE

Within every Indian household, there lies a masala (spice) dhaba (container). Now if you own one of these, you have officially obtained the 'aunty or uncle' status. This is a round container made of steel; and in that container, will be one cylindrical small bowl surrounded by six of the same bowls. Each one has it's own spice. These are the every day, staple spices used in cooking. They create a perfect balance. So much so, that we can relate these spices to the essential components of our happiness. If I had to select seven 'spices' that would lead to happiness, it would include the following:

1. Gratitude: feel it every day. It doesn't always have to be major. It can be for the simplest of things that we sometimes take for granted, like clean water that is readily available for us to drink, or the ability to pick up the phone and call someone who we miss.

2. Forgiveness: it's a litte more difficult, this one. But it can be accomplished once you put your mind to it. Harboring negative feelings and holding on to anger and resentment will only do more harm to you than the person you have these feelings for. So best is to let it go.

3. Empathy: Be able to understand, without judgement, what someone else may be going through. It give us more perspective and helps us to be less reactive.

4. Contribution: Do something nice without expecting something in return. It does not have to be a huge deal.

Simple small acts. Hold the door, smile, say hello, help someone with their bags. You will feel good, and it will greatly affect the other person's day. You don't realize the impact you may have on someone's life with just a moment of time. Why not make it a positive one?

5. Be less serious: We were all kids one time, and somewhere along the lines we grew up and forgot that silliness is OK. We started to care what people think and how we 'should' behave. Laugh hard, dance around, have FUN, and let loose. My mom is naturally this way, and I am lucky to have her around, because we can be so silly with one another- it keeps us young at heart.

6. Positive thinking: Approach each day, each project, each problem, with a positive outlook. What's the alternative? Might as well walk in with an optimistic and confident attitude, because that may have an uplifting effect on

others, and in turn, will help solve matters efficiently and more effectively. Never underestimate the power of positive thinking.

7. Self love: I would put this one as the central spice; for obvious reasons.

THE SMILE FACTOR

When you're upset, depressed, or angry, someone may tell you to "cheer up and smile." At that point, you look at them in awe – thinking of their audacity to say this to you. You secretly want to take a frying pan and hit them on their cheery-ass head, and knock that stupid smile off their face. Yes, we've ALL been there.

Unfortunately, as it always does, science wins here. It has been proven that this simple act of allowing your facial muscles to form a smile can lift your spirits, lower stress, and increase your immune system. Crazy? I know. You can "trick" your brain into believing you're happy, just by smiling (even if you really have no desire to smile). If you smile more, your mood will improve, and you will send more positive vibes to the people around you. When you smile, your brain releases "feel-good" neurotransmitters, which aid in calming your nervous system.

Your smile is a powerful tool – for yourself and for others around you. Can someone really be offended by your smile? Your simple act of smiling can actually change his/her entire day. In turn, they may smile at someone else, because now THEY are happy because YOU smiled at them. So, see what you have created here? A domino smile. How beautiful is that?

If you're reading this and rolling your eyes, or if you're reading this at all, just do it. Smile. Put a big, warm smile on your face. Think of someone who you love, and you are seeing them after a long period of time. Now think of something negative, but KEEP smiling. It's hard to hold on to that negative thought, isn't it?

Smiling doesn't make you WEAK, or less "manly," nor does it diminish whatever 'powerful' status you're trying to hold on to. People actually want to be around others who are generally positive and who smile more. What a concept! Positive, smiling people, will attract positive, smiling people, and these are exactly the types of people with whom you want to surround yourself. So if you're a mopey, negative, "Debbie Downer," get out of that funk, put on a smile, and know that you're not the only one in a bad funk. No one will truly help you but yourself in terms of getting into a good mental state. So, when you dress yourself every day, don't forget to wear the most important accessory – your SMILE.

PS: Have you heard of laughter therapy? Yes, it's a big thing. Google it. It works.

I'M TOO SEXY FOR MYSELF

A very, very, very close individual to me was going through a separation, just one year after I packed my bags and left California. I sometimes think that the universe sent me back so I could hold her hand through it. She had just had her first born child, and found out that her husband was having an affair. Combine that with post-partum. OUCH. She was in a bad, bad place. And, at that point, I could not just tell her to "be positive and smile." Are you kidding me? She would probably chop me into pieces and shoot me down the garbage disposal and wave good-bye <with a smile on her face, of course>. And it would have been a very insensitive piece of advice to give.

The best I could do was to give her space so she could feel her emotions, go through the grieving process, and I would be there to listen. I stayed with her a few nights out of the week and we spent a lot of time together. One year went by and she was getting stronger by the day, but still had her moments of loneliness. When I thought she may be ready to start socializing, I demanded (yes, it's good to be demanding at times) that we both dress up and go out. I bought a bunch of sexy outfits for her, we got our eyebrows done together (Indian women and eyebrows are not friends –- let's just put it that way), and we felt great, Like we were free from all negativity. From that evening onward, we were painting the town red and enjoying our lives. We were in a state of "happy," even though we didn't have the most ideal situations. You can still be happy if everything in your life is not perfect. It's most definitely possible.

I want to emphasize the importance of looking good for YOURSELF. Whatever you feel that defines your physical appearance, do it. Everyone has his/her own take on what looks "good," or "sexy." If you're going to sulk in despair, not bathe, wear the same jeans you have been wearing for 4 days, you will feel gloomy inside (and no one will want to hang out with you because you probably stink). So how you feel on the outside definitely affects how you feel on the inside. Give yourself time to heal from emotional wounds; but if you give yourself TOO much time, it may become a "downward spiral" situation. **Dwelling on what went wrong will not make things right.** Understanding that you went through some tough shit, grieving over it to get it out of your system, and moving on to make the right choices so that you do not end up in that state again, is the only way you will be able to embrace what the future holds for you. And that future is all dependent on your state of mind. Your state of mind will dictate your daily routine. Your state of mind will dictate the people with whom you choose to connect. Your state of mind will dictate YOU. Feeling sexy only physically will not do the trick; you must feel it emotionally as well. Sexy is a state of mind. Wear it and feel it.

IT'S NEVER TOO LATE TO CHANGE

YOUR STORY

Everyone comes into this world with his/her own story and their own experiences. We have the ability to shape our lives with the decisions we make. Either we can allow our past situations to loom over our future like a gray, sad cloud, or we can take those experiences and say "FUCK YOU, you are not going to dictate the rest of my remaining years."

Learn from them, lift yourself up from them, rise above them, and understand that we all have bad experiences — some are greater or lesser levels of "bad," but, at the end of the day, how you let them shape your future is KEY. And it's up to YOU. You determine that. You can choose to get out of your head, and make your life story count; not for anyone else, but for yourself. Do it for YOU. There is a road to happiness, but we need to actively take the steps to get there, and we have all the tools necessary to do so.

The time for happy is NOW. Not I'll be happy "when," but I'll be happy NOW. Enjoy the journey that life brings to us, instead of waiting for some "pot of gold" that is expected at the end. Take notice of the treasures that you have every day right in front of you, and understand that the fact that you are alive and breathing is one of the most remarkable experiences ever. Make the life that we are given one in which we can look back on with genuine smiles on our faces, knowing that we played our cards to the best of our abilities; one in which we became the best versions of ourselves that we could possibly be; and one in which we made a positive difference or two, in the lives of others. Let's be grateful for the life we have been gifted. Let's start making a positive shift in our thoughts, and understand that happiness is a state of mind, a feeling over which we have complete control.

About the Author

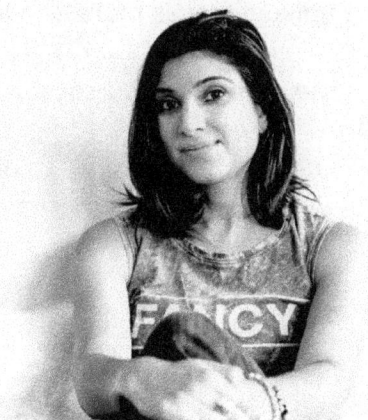

Photo Credit : Angie Trowbridge

Born and raised in Rocky Mount, North Carolina, Pooja is the second daughter of Indian-born parents who immigrated to the United States in 1975 in hopes to start a new life. Her parents are her inspiration and she is grateful for their presence every day.

She obtained her Bachelor of Science degree in Civil Engineering with a minor in Psychology from The George Washington University in Washington, DC, and currently does absolutely nothing with that degree; however, the experience of the university was more of a lesson in many aspects of life. She currently pursues her passion in interior and event decor and operates a company known as Amoda Decor; Amod meaning "happy" in Sanskrit, as she followed her happiness, and advises everyone to do the same, whatever it may be.

She is happily married and blessed with three adorable girls. To her, grateful is an understatement.

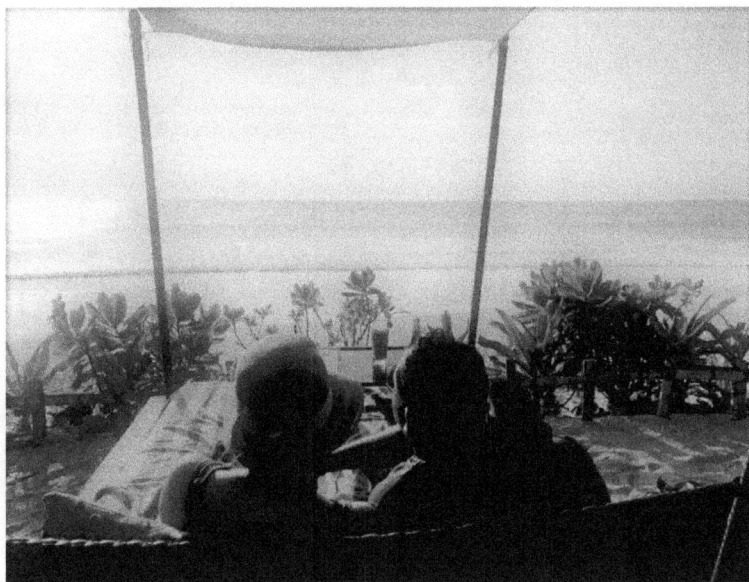

www.ingramcontent.com/pod-product-compliance
Lightning Source LLC
Chambersburg PA
CBHW031131020426
42333CB00012B/319